How To Lose 23 Pounds Of Fat Without Torture Diets Or Hard Exercise And Keep It Off(The Compass Method)

Dr. Chio Ugochukwu

Published by Compass International

44546 Orchard Lane, Lancaster CA 93534

ISBN-13: 978-1517120627

ISBN-10: 1517120624

Printed in the United States of America

Table of Contents

Introduction

There are many different reasons for losing weight and keeping it off. The reasons range from health and medical reasons like diabetes, sleeping and breathing problems to social reasons like being more active and having more fun.

Losing weight is also important because obesity affects a large number of people. According to Koebnick et al (2012) in a study of about 1.8 million young adults aged 20 to 39 years, 29.9% of young adults are obese while about 6.1% of women and 4.5% of men have extreme obesity. The Robert Wood Johnson Foundation spends about $500 million dollars every year trying to stop the increase or occurrence of childhood obesity (Anshel, 2010).

According to the CDC more than 34% of

adults in America are obese. Obesity is common, expensive to manage and can be deadly because of its association with health-related conditions like stroke, diabetes and heart disease which are among the leading causes of death in the united States. About 300,000 people die every year in America from obesity-related health problems (Samaranayake, Ong, Leung & Chueng, 2012).

Sadly, though most people are aware of the dangers or consequences of being overweight, including its association with reduced quality of life, few people are able to consistently implement those steps that will enable them lose weight and keep it off. According to Ansel (2010) though most people believe that exercise is good for their health, 60-70% of adults who start a health-related program stop the program within 6-9months. Part of the reason why this happens is that most people with the intention to improve their health try to make major changes to their lifestyle, without a better understanding of themselves, their motivations, and what will work best for them as individuals.

Through this book, I will share with you some of the most effective and easy to implement ways you can make significant and individualized changes to your lifestyle that will help you lose weight and keep it off. This can be done as a step by step process through the Compass Method. First, I will give you the outline of the Compass Method, then I will share details and examples that will help you apply this holistic approach to yourself.

The Compass Method For Losing Weight And Keeping It Off

This is an outline of the Compass Method that shows you the simple steps you can take to make the lifestyle adjustments that will help you reduce your weight and keep it off. The first step in this process is to learn more about yourself so that you will have the mind-set that will help you to take effective daily action, instead of continually looking for a single magical solution.

Even in nature, it is self-evident that simple solutions are the most enduring. They are fun to do and lead to more consistent results. **This is why the Compass Method for losing weight is based on the following simple steps:**

1, Know yourself better.

This will help your adjust your mindset, and become more confident in the decisions you make and the actions you take. Without confidence in yourself, you will be prone to too many decision reversals and over reliance on other people's opinion.

2, Know your personality

Though no one definition of personality is universally accepted, your personality is generally accepted to mean the pattern of relatively permanent traits and unique characteristics that gives both consistency and individuality to the way you behave or function in different circumstances and situations (Feist & Feist, 2009). With this definition in mind, you can see why it will be important for you to make understanding your personality an important part of your individualized weight-loss plan.

3, Adjust your diet

4, Reduce stress

You will learn about how to do this in this book and cut down on using food or eating as a coping mechanism for stress management and build on your strengths.

5, Improve your daily emotional well being

6, Maintain your balance

7, Do daily consistent exercise

8, Manage your finances

9, Work with a group

10, Review, Adjust and Persist (RAP)

Through the rest of this book, I will share with you in more details how you can craft your own individualized weight-loss plan through the use of the Compass Method. We shall begin the process by learning about how you can use the compass profiles to influence your strategy for weight loss.

How to use the compass profiles to understand yourself better and facilitate your weight loss

The compass health profiles are the foundation for the compass method for transformational living. You can apply the method to your weight loss strategy. Here are the components of the compass profile.

Compass Health Profiles:

C = Community Relationships.

O = Operational capacity profile.

M= Metabolic profile.

P= Physical profile.

A= Ambition profile.

S= Spiritual profile.

S = Self Knowledge profile.

How do you use these profiles to help you lose weight, improve your health, and transform your life? According to current medical research those who have good **relationships** with themselves, their family and their friends tend to live longer and healthier lives. **This is part of the community relationships profile.**

The first step in relating to others is relating to yourself. Communicate with yourself first and write down your deepest fears and worries. What is holding you back from talking to others? What is affecting your confidence in yourself and your ability to make decisions? What is holding you back from making a commitment to change yourself? Is it fear of the process or fear of communication?

Good communication is good because it helps to reduce stress. If you feel you are not good at it, don't let it bother you. Do the best you can do. The smallest action is better than the greatest intention. Taking action will help you reduce stress and have more energy for all the fun things you would like to do with your life. Nothing in life is perfect, so if you find some of these steps too hard to take, begin with the actions you can take today.

Answering or asking these questions, will help you recognize which aspects of your relationship with others could either be contributing to your weight gain or making it more difficult for you to lose weight. Just remember that you can also make your friends part of your family. After all, good companionship from those we live with and interact with everyday, helps us live to longer and better. This requires a lot of give and take.

Through your **operational capacity profile,** you will learn how to analyze things for yourself, how to get things done and how you can continue to improve. The simplest way to do this is to look back at your life and find out which method of preparation and execution has worked the best for you in your most successful projects. You can then modify your weight-loss strategy to fit that model.

Include in your project review, things like getting ready for vacations, birthday parties or getting ready for a wedding or tasks as simple as going to work on time and cleaning your house. For most people, the best way to tackle most projects is to start on time and break them down into small simple steps. For others every project is eventually done at the last minute.

If you like to get things done at the last minute, it means you tend to procrastinate and underestimate how much time you would need to get things done. Remember that inadequate preparation leads to failure. To lose weight and keep it off, you will have to start with a small plan and build on it slowly, in a way that suits your internal and external circumstances.

Your **Metabolic profile** will include both your nutritional and metabolic analysis. You can get your metabolic analysis by getting your physiological and laboratory tests done. This will help you to know if there are significant medical problems responsible for your weight. Getting the right tests done with the help of a healthcare professional or your doctor will make it easy for you to know which aspect of your health profile you need to focus on improving.

When it comes to losing weight even without running tests, **your family history can help you a get a better** picture of your risk factors. If you have a family history of diabetes or chronic obesity, then you have to be much more vigilant than others.

The Physical Profile includes your weight, height, waist circumference and BMI(Body Mass Index). It also includes your heart rate and lung function. These factors are important because it is important to know your health status before you can engage in vigorous exercise. **Take action today, weigh yourself today, even if you feel you are in excellent health.**

The main exercise protocol proposed in **the Compass Method** is mild to moderate activities like **walking**, dancing, jump ropes and pushups. If you are more used to vigorous exercise like playing basketball, tennis, and baseball, you need to remember to check with their doctor to make sure that you are healthy enough to continue to exercise vigorously. One advantage of staying physically active is that it helps you burn off excessive energy that would have been converted to fat. Increased storage of excess energy in the form of fat will ultimately build up your weight and cause more health problems.

The Ambition profile looks at your job and finances and satisfaction with your life. This is important because without good finances or insurance it is much more difficult to take good care of your health. The ambition profile measures your ability to get things done or to make adjustments when they are required. **Set measurable goals like reducing your weight by 10Lbs. This is an important bench mark because once you can confidently write down the actions and activities that helped you lose your first 10 pounds, you can build on it to lose more pounds.**

The remaining two profiles are **Spirituality and Self Knowledge**, both of which examine your psychospiritual make up. They will help you have a **better understanding of your personality,** character and connection with God and the universe. **Knowing your personality type will give you a greater insight into how personality affects your weight loss strategy.** Though there are many classifications or names for different personality types, **the DISC personality profile is the one used in the Compass Method.**

A better understanding of your psychological strengths and weaknesses will help you know your limitations, when it comes to choosing pathways to better health. It will also help you to anticipate problems, quarrels and pressure points.

On the spiritual side of the equation, more and more studies are beginning to show that those who meditate or are truly prayerful are better able to handle health challenges than those who do neither. Of course I realize that there are different interpretations of what it means to be spiritual and that one size does not fit all. Next we shall begin the whole process by finding out how your passion can affect your weight-loss strategy.

Assignment

Write down a paragraph that best explains your best understanding of yourself, including your strengths and weaknesses

How to use your passion to lose weight

If you really want to lose weight you have to make your passion work for you. Knowing your passion is part of how you know yourself. This is because unless you have a better understanding of yourself, you will always stumble or have difficulty as you try to relate to others and to yourself.

Your passion is part of what connects you to the world. What one thing or item would you like to change in the world? Your answer here could be a multitude of things including providing better drinking water, helping underprivileged children or helping to stop the extinction of an animal. The point is that if you do not stay healthy by losing weight, you will not be able to follow your passion. This is why you have to make getting motivated by your passion the cornerstone of your individualized plan to lose weight.

You can also discover you passion by asking yourself relevant questions about what you like to do in your spare time. You probably spend time doing things you are passionate about. You may spend time hiking, writing, playing music, exercising or doing whatever you enjoy.

What makes you smile? All those things that make you smile are things that you love and enjoy doing. Of course, it doesn't have to be an item. Spending time with your grandchildren or visiting a senior home can be other things that put a smile on your face.

Go through this list and start writing down your answers. From here you want to see if there is one thing that gets repeated again and again. If so, chances are that this is your passion.

By finding your passion and making it a greater part of your life, you will enjoy more of your daily activities and cut down on stress. This will help you reduce the tendency to eat snacks to cope with daily emotional pains. I know I have had to frequently deal with this problem myself until I finally came to accept my passion and the challenges that are associated with it.

The good thing to remember is that after sometime, you probably have a good idea about your passion, your strengths and weaknesses. Focus more on your strengths and take daily action to enjoy your hobbies and interests. **Take action that will help your talents and gifts flourish instead of worrying about your weaknesses and what negative people have to say about you.**

The more you use your passion to focus on the positive, the less stressed out you will be. The less stressed out you are, the less you will be tempted to use eating as a way to cope with your emotional challenges. The more you can manage or control what you eat the more you can lose weight in a sustainable way. Next you need to learn about how your personality can affect your weight-loss strategy.

Assignment

Ask questions that will help you discover your passion

Make your passion the anchor reason why you want to lose weight

Find out your personality type

How to take advantage of a deeper understanding of your personality in your weight-loss strategy

Though your personality can play a significant role on how much weight you lose and how much weight you keep off, a lot of people do not consider it when trying to lose weight. Part of the reason for this is that most people cannot see the relationship between their weight and their personalities. The other reason could be because there are many different personality types with different confusing explanations.

I used to find them quite confusing until, I learned about the DISC personality types. The "D" personality or choleric is demanding, decisive, loves pressure, and being in control. If you love structure and being in control then make your individualized weight-loss plan such that it includes a written plan with specific daily meal preferences. The best way to do this would be to write down your specific fruits and nuts choices **after your 72-hour meal audit**. You would also benefit from a detailed weekly journal through which you write down the type of food you ate, or plan to eat, your food portions, with a record of your calories in and out.

On the other hand if you are an "I" personality or sanguine, you will find detailed journal writing unbearable because you do not enjoy details and only prefer broad outlines for your weight-loss strategy. The danger is that as an outgoing person you may sometimes find yourself so short of time, that you may begin to rely too much on processed food to meet your energy needs. The solution is to plan ahead and keep things simple and easily adjustable. You may also find it more helpful to be part of a support group that will help you to remain disciplined and follow through with your weight-loss strategy and avoid distractions.

If you are a "C" dominant personality or melancholy or beavers, then you will love explanations, time to think and details. Journaling may work for you, and you are more likely to find regular reading of nutrition facts helpful in forming your own individualized weight-loss strategy. However do not fall into analysis paralysis, where you spend so much time looking for the perfect and most precise weight-loss plan for yourself as an individual that you never get started. Begin with the best information and ideas that you have. Remember that as a "C" your basic motivation is quality and correctness while the basic motivation of the "D" is challenge and control.

If your personality type is "S" or phlegmatic or golden retrievers, you have to remember that you are motivated by support and stability, and are averse to risk taking. This means you may be more interested in making the food you are already used to eating more healthy and weight-loss appropriate than in trying new exotic meals or new ways of exercising. This means that your most effective weight-loss strategy might come from calorie reduction or keeping a close eye on the food you eat and making your daily exercise more efficient.

On the other hand an "I" dominant personality type who loves to be recognized and loves taking risks, might be more interested in more exotic healthy meals and participating in group exercises and adventures. The bottom line is you have to remember that your personality will influence your basic motivations for participating in different aspects of your daily life. This is why you have to take your personality type into consideration when crafting or implementing your own individualized weight-loss strategy through the Compass Method. Next you need to learn to make adjustments to your daily meal instead of trying to learn a new diet every six months.

Assignment

Find out more about how personality type contributes to your daily choices and decisions

If you want to learn more about your

DISC personality visit;

http://www.compasswellnessinstitute.com/your-disc-personality-profile/

How to adjust your diet and lose weight

The problem most people have is that they get so caught up with trying new ways of eating healthy that they keep on changing plans. This is like trying to build a house without ever getting past choosing the design.

Instead of torturing yourself by chasing the latest complicated diet fad, adjust what you eat everyday to what is healthy and enjoyable to you. This is part of the Compass Method, because we believe it will be easier to make adjustments to the food you are used to eating than to try to acquire a new taste. Most people that begin a new diet find it hard to sustain and end up quitting before they can see tangible results.

The first step to take would be to cut down the servings or portions of your regular meal by

half. This will reduce your energy intake by about half or a third. You fill the gap with vegetables and fruits. If you feel pangs of hunger, snack with nuts, drink plenty of water or eat some fruits.

The more your servings are reduced, the more weight you would lose because the fewer calories you will take in, the more energy will be obtained from excess body fat resulting in weight loss. However, reduced servings may mean more hunger pangs. This is a serious potential problem that sometimes makes people drink a lot of soda or eat many hot dogs as an immediate way of dealing with their hunger pangs. This simply leads to more energy intake and more weight gain.

To deal with this, eat more fruits, vegetables and fibers as fillers. Fibers are especially good for your system because they help to increase bowel movement. This has the added effect of making your digestive system more efficient.

For different cultures and settings, different modifications to familiar eating habits can be made. In America this would entail cutting down on fast foods, soda and other processed foods. You can do this by going to eat fast food only once a month. If you cannot do this, start by either eating only small sizes or eating only half of the sandwich that you buy.

Do not go along with food choices that will not be good for your health just because people from your culture may challenge you or make fun of you. Your culture is supposed to help you, not to kill you. You can do this by finding a way to eat right within your culture.

Do a 72-hour food audit before you make the final decision on your adjustments. You can do this by simply writing down the food, drinks and snacks you have eaten in the past 72 hours. Through your food audit, you will know what food dominates your eating pattern and what adjustments you need to make. When I did my food audit, I found out that my eating pattern was dominated by rice and bread. I made changes. I added more, corn, fruits and nuts to my daily food.

I also found out through my food audit that while my goal was to reduce sodium intake to about 1500 mg per day and cut down my energy intake by half. The challenge to this goal was that while I was able to quickly reduce my food portions, I found myself snacking too much everyday. I was eating about 10 slices of bread everyday. This meant I was already getting too much sodium and calories just from bread alone without even adding my other sources of sodium. On the average a slide of bread contains 150 mg of sodium and 110 calories per serving. This would mean that for bread with one slice per serving, 10 slices would be 1100calories. This would be more than the average 2000 calories per day recommended for most people.

Finally, I figured out why despite my reduction in portions, regular exercise and eating fruits and vegetables my weight loss was slow and inconsistent. To make matters worse, I had been using nuts for snacks without checking their sugar content and calories per serving. One small pack of unsalted pea nuts contained 220 calories per serving but 6 servings per pack. How does this information which I read from the nutrition facts on the pack help?

Here is how it helps. When I finish a pack of pea nuts which was rich in dietary fiber, with little or zero sodium and cholesterol, I was also eating (6x220=1320) calories. When you combine it with my 10 slices of bread with 1100 calories, it means that from bread and peanuts alone, I had already eaten (1100+1320=2420) calories.

This shows that though I had reduced my calories per meal through reducing my portion per meal, because I had not paid careful attention to size or frequency of my snacks, I was eating a lot of calories per day through snacks. As soon as I discovered this, I cut my snack portions by half and cut down my slices of bread to, not more than 4 per day. This helped me reduce my extra calories by more than half. This adjustment helped me to start losing weight more consistently and keeping it off. **If you want to lose fat, you have to know your daily sources of extra calories.**

You do not have to do this type of detailed estimate of your energy intake to know your average energy intake. All you have to do is to remember that you have to reduce all sources of

your daily intake of calories from your meals to your snacks. Do this to a level that allows you to feel full, eat healthy and still lose weight.

According to surveys by doctors and nutritionists the average American male takes about 3,000 calories per day and the female 2,400 calories per day (Reuters Health, 2015). According to Dr. Wang an energy intake and expenditure expert, consistent loss or reduction in energy intake of 100 calories would lead to 10 pounds loss in weight (Reuters Health, 2015). **This means that without knowing the exact quantity of calories you eat, you can continue to reduce your meal, snack or social eating portions until you notice your first loss of 10 pounds and use it for a marker or foundation for all your future weight-loss strategies.**

Apart from the reduction in food portion, I also started drinking a glass of water before each meal. This helped me feel full, without eating as much as before. After a while, I was able to consistently cut down my slices of bread to 2 to 4, instead of 10. As a result my sodium intake and calorie intake reduced.

The good news is that this approach is not unique to me. You too can do this. Research has shown that drinking water before a meal will help to expand your stomach. This approach will make you feel completely full when you are only 80% full. This is important because eating only up to 80 % full was one of the common practices of people of Okinawa in Japan, who have the highest number of centenarians in the world (Boyle & Long, 2010). My suggestion is that you drink at least two glasses of water per meal and increase the bulk in your meals through fruits and vegetables. **This will**

help you reduce your total calorie intake per meal without tortures diets.

To increase my intake of fruits and vegetables, I started eating every rice meal with salads consisting of cabbage, tomatoes, carrots, broccoli, spinach and bananas. Eating a colorful variety of fruits and vegetables per meal with reduced portions of brown rice made my meal significantly more healthy and more bulky but less energy dense. It has helped me to lose significant pounds and keep them off. I am sure that if you do the same, your meals will become more healthy and less energy dense. **Remember calories in calories out.**

You need to be careful when you start cutting down on calories by reducing the intake of carbohydrate like white bread, white rice or pasta. This will make you lose weight quickly because it is usually stored in the body as glycogen which contains water. You need to be careful because the brain gets most of its energy from glucose and if it does not get enough you begin to feel tired, weak, unable to sleep and ill. Unless you switch to fiber-rich carbohydrate sources like baked sweet potato, whole grain bread, barley, oat meal and brown rice, you may end up quitting after a few weeks. This is why **the Compass Method is focused on adjustments and individualized modifications**.

Whatever you decide, start small. Remember that little drops of water make the mighty ocean. This thought will help you, even when you feel overwhelmed by the thought of changing your eating habits. When I changed my eating habits, I started by making small changes like adding salads to every meal of rice that I had. I found the whole idea difficult initially but I had to remind myself the passion behind my decision to lose weight. Try a few combinations to find out what will work best for you.

To make sustainable adjustments and modifications to your meals concentrate on variety and moderation. Include chicken, fish, beans, cottage cheese, or low fat yogurt in your meals. Have eggs, nuts and red meat occasionally. You can further reduce your fat intake by eating skinless chicken or turkey. Turkey and chicken have their fat on their skin but red meat has most of its fat contained within the meat. Grilling is better than frying, and always aim to use unsaturated oils like corn, and olive oils for cooking.

You can also gradually reduce the fat content in your milk products. You can do this by changing from whole milk, to 2% fat; then to 1% fat. We do not recommend fat free milk because it is important to get fat in your body which can be used through cellular metabolism to produce cell membranes and hormones. Choose lower-fat cheese and yogurt. When you buy yogurt, also check that it does not contain sugar. The good thing about reducing to 1% fat milk is that it remains tasteful. Fat has 9 calories of energy per gram compared to carbohydrate and proteins that have about 4 per gram.

Remember that variety is the spice of life.
Do not eat the same meal day in day out. Why? It gets boring after a while and you will soon find yourself looking less forward to eating healthy.
Make sure your food contains **adequate** but moderate portions of fat, proteins, carbohydrates and vitamins. Eat enough food to fill full, when you eat. If you don't fill full after a meal you will find yourself eating too much sugary snacks in between meals to make you feel full. This will

make you gain back weight you may have lost. If you feel hungry between meals, snack with small portions of almonds, cashew nuts or peanuts. Almonds will make you feel less hungry and still boost your metabolism.

Eat everything in moderation. Do not eat a particular food too much just because you like it. This was like how I used to a lot of white bread and soda just because, I liked them. Concentrate on eating non-processed food instead of on processed food like bacon and "ready-to-go" meals like frozen burritos and pizzas. They are convenient but have high sugar and high dense calories!

Be particularly careful with how much soda or beer you drink. Beer has a lot of calories with little ingredients. Drinking too much beer may cost you some important vitamins like vitamin B 6. Another way to balance your meal would be to halve your intake of all pure or added fats as previously outlined.

Plan your meals and snacks ahead of time. Take time to plan at least one lunch and dinner every week without meat or cheese. Build those meals around whole grains, vegetables and beans to increase fiber and reduce fat. If you want to have something to chew on, get some fish or tofu. You can make every Friday your fish meal day.

Have at least five servings of fruit every day. This can be for dessert or snacks. Choose fruit that is in season. My rule is to take an apple per meal. If you can, go for those red delicious apples because they contain pectin, a fiber that helps to promote healthy cholesterol levels and contain more amounts of antioxidants than many other types of apples.

Assignment

Do your 72-hour food audit

Cut down your serving portions for meals

Eat food that is rich in fruits and whole grains

Modify your typical cultural food

Drink two glasses of water before every meal

Eat an apple per meal

Plan your snacks in advance

Cut down on your snack portions

Cut down on soda and beer

Make reading your nutritional facts part of your strategy to lose weight and keep it off

You have to look at reading your nutritional facts the same way you look at reading or looking at your gas or fuel gauge in your car. If you do not form the habit of checking your gas gauge in your car, you could end up with an empty tank in the middle of nowhere or in a very dangerous part of town.

Reading your nutritional facts will give you an idea of the quantity, food types and ingredients in the food you eat everyday. This will help you know how much calories, carbohydrate, fat, protein and sodium is in the food you eat. Physiologically sodium which is the main component of salt draws in water wherever it is found in the body. This means that if you do not watch your total sodium intake, you may unwittingly expose yourself to daily fluctuations in your weight, depending on how much water you retain.

This usually happens because other sources of sodium have not been accounted for. This includes salt used in cooking and salt used in preserving pre-cooked food. The first is obvious while the second will involve some research. Unfortunately, most of us do not have time for research so we just end up eating with sounds healthy and move on.

The problem is that without taking the time to read our nutritional labels we could end up eating more fluid-retaining-food or food high in calories without knowing it. This was what happened to a Jane, a 42-year old woman, who had been trying to lose weight. She had been doing well, losing weight as planned, until she hit a bump in her weight-loss journey. She stopped losing weight and started gaining weight though she had kept everything about the same in her life. Later, it turned out that about a week before she had changed her shift at her job. She now had to leave the house much earlier, so as a temporary solution, she started eating *Green Burritos* for breakfast on her way to work.

Her problem was resolved, when at my urging she did her own 72-hour food audit and realized that the burrito was the only difference to her food menu in the past few weeks. When she finally took the time to read the nutrition label, she discovered that the "Green Burrito", she had thought was healthy, contained about 1200 mg of sodium per serving. She quickly stopped eating it and her weight gain stopped.

Do you know how much salt is contained in pre-cooked burrito? On average one burrito has 470mg to 1200mg of sodium. These are significant numbers especially, if you are trying to keep your daily sodium intake to 1500mg of sodium or less. For, Jane this meant that with two serving of her large burrito, she would have accumulated 2400 mg of sodium. This means that by the end of the day from lunch, supper and other snacks she could be well within 3000mg of sodium daily. This will make her retain a lot of water and gain weight. You could be doing the same to yourself, if you do not watch your sodium intake by taking time to read your nutrition facts.

Generally, when I look at my nutrition facts, I look at my sodium, potassium, fiber, sugar, calories and fat content. I know people sometimes ignore their sodium content, thinking it does not really matter. Well, it does. When comparing a loaf of bread with a can of soda, you will find that on average a single serving of bread contains 150 milligrams of sodium, while the can of soda contains 65 milligrams of sodium per serving size.

The other important facts you will learn about the food you are about to eat by looking at the food label, would be how much sugar it has, and the calories per serving. This is important because you need to cut down you calorie intake to lose weight. Studies have shown that it is easier to lose weight by reducing energy intake, than by trying to use exercise and physical activity to burn off excess energy intake after eating too much. **Unless you get this principle clear and apply it daily to your weight loss strategies, you will fail. This is the principle of calories in, calories out**.

If you enjoy eating bread because of its fibers you may unwittingly be eating too much sodium or eating sugar. A serving of bread, which is usually one or two slices, also contains on average 3g of sugar. According to the American Heart Association (AHA), the recommended sugar intake for men is 37.5g and for women 25g. This means that if you eat 8 servings of bread, you would have eaten 24g of sugar. The increase in sugar in your body can lead to an increase in your triglycerides and lead to a reduction in the level of high density lipoproteins (HDL) in your body.

By reading your food facts you will know how much sodium or sugar each choice you make will add to your daily energy intake. All you need is a broad idea, you do not need to count calories or know the percentage daily value of everything you eat. This type of knowledge will ultimately help you to control or reduce your total calories without putting too much effort into it.

The more you know about the daily factors that can affect your weight, and take action, the more you will be able to eat healthy in a smart way that works for you, without getting on torture diets. Next you have to acquire the habit of eating slowly.

Assignment

Start reading your nutrition facts regularly

Cut down on your total sodium intake and not just added salt

Cut down on your daily sugar intake

Stop the mistake of eating your food too fast if you want to lose weight and keep it off

Sadly most of us are so busy that we have to repeatedly do more than one thing at a time. Even if you did all the modifications to make your daily meals healthy but ended up eating fast, you will end up over eating. Eat slowly. The body is slow to register when you are full and it is easy to eat too much if you are racing through your meals. You can easily do this if you eat and do other things at the same time.

Eating and watching TV. If you eat and watch TV you do not pay as much attention as you should to your food so you end up eating fast and shoveling your food down your throat. Try as much as you can to switch off the TV when you eat. That includes snacks as well as meals. Studies have proved that we eat larger portions in front of the TV, probably because we are much less aware of what we are eating.

According to Cleland, Schmidt, Dwyer, &Venn, (2008) time spent in behaviors that involve a lot of sitting with little activity, like watching or viewing TV was thought to be one of the factors responsible for increasing number of people that either overweight or obese in different parts of the world. The study also found that in both men and women the average time spent watching television increased with the increasing frequency of consuming food and drinks while watching television. Soft drink consumption during television viewing was associated with a greater increase in abdominal obesity in both men and women.

Eating and working is another habit that makes you eat your food in a hurry instead of slowly. This is a very common practice among handy men. They pick up their hamburgers and chew on them while they hammer nails into the wall. Two problems here are poor digestion and more accidents or injuries. Give one activity your full attention, then move on to the next.

Choose food that you can chew. Again this will increase your fiber intake, and the act of chewing will make you feel more satisfied too. This means eating fruit instead of drinking juice. If you have soup, make sure it is chunky.

Another way you can get yourself to eat more slowly and enjoy your food more is to find a place where you eat on a regular basis everyday. This could be eating breakfast at home, instead of in your car. If due to your busy schedule you cannot do this in the morning then make it your super. **Instead of sitting in front of the TV after work , eating and watching TV, sit at your dining table and eat your super slowly. Next take care of conversational stress.**

Assignment

**Stop eating and watching TV at the same time
Do one at a time**

Avoid making the mistake of taking conversational stress for granted when you are trying to lose weight

Your daily conversations are an important part of your daily life. It is through them that you relate to friends, family and co-workers. It can also be a source of stress and anxiety.

Coping with conversational stress is important because we interact with others through our conversations with them. We do this by listening to others, talking to others and responding to what others say or have failed to say or do. Unless we are able to make the distinction between what needs a response what does not, we may end up getting worked up.

A simple strategy for coping with the potential emotional tension that may sometimes arise from our daily conversations would be to divide our conversations or activities into "little rocks" and "heavy rocks". Little rocks are those conversations you can either overlook or can decide to ignore without losing out significantly. What is an example of little rock conversation? If you are in the midst of a conversation with your brother and he is arguing that the sun goes round the earth, what will you say? Will you continue to argue even when you have shown him irrevocable evidence and he continues to argue? Arguing for arguing sake will only get you worked up and build up your stress level. This is an example of the "Little rocks" in a conversation. Let it go! **You don't have to have the last word.**

If you do not let it go, stress will build up and lead to the release of hormones that will make you store more fat. Corticosteroids which are released by the adrenal gland during stress can lead to increase in belly fat.

You have more important things to do with your time and energy than getting into conversations that do not enhance your sense of well-being. **Instead learn to focus on your main goals in each conversational encounter. Ignore those who like to put you down on get into quarrels and point making.**

Create time to take care of your daily "big rocks". Spending quality time with your family should be considered a 'big rock". You could go and watch a movie with your friend, wife or partner. You could go swimming or go for a walk in the park. You could spend more time working on projects or goals that mean a lot to you. Next focus on ways to increase your daily physical activity.

Assignment

You do not have to have the last word

Make increased physical activity part of your daily strategy for losing weight and keeping it off

You need to make a conscious effort to increase your daily physical activity. This would include deliberately looking for ways to participate in physical activities at home. You could decide to mow the lawn yourself instead of giving out as a contract to others. You could also participate more in gardening or yard cleaning, every little bit counts. Remember that little drops of water make the mighty ocean.

Increased daily physical activity has the metabolic effect of helping you burn off energy everyday, so that there is less excess energy left in the body to be converted to fat for storage. The less fat you store, the more fat you would lose.

You can also increase physical activity by doing something as simple as walking to as many places as you can everyday. As you go through your daily activities, make it a point to walk a little further. One of my favorite tricks for doing this is to park far away from the entrance each time I go to the grocery store or the mall. This will help you take a few more steps everyday. Try it. You will be surprised at how effective this can become for you without changing your lifestyle a great deal.

There are several different exercises or physical activities that you can do to help you burn off more energy and minimize the effects of daily stress in your life. Walking is among the best, as you can easily lose yourself and your troubles by walking. Even if it is just around the block, walking can do wonders for your health. It can also help to reduce your stress level.

If you have a lot of stress in your life, you may want to consider a gym or doing yoga stretches at home. Working out and then sitting in the sauna is also a good way to relieve tension. It will also help you sweat a lot and lose more weight. First you have to make sure you are healthy enough by asking your doctor if you can use a sauna.

If you do not like walking or going to the gym, consider going for swimming exercises, joining a dance class or even playing tennis. If you have a pool at home, you may find swimming to be very beneficial way to increase physical activity and help you relax.

If you find yourself doing a lot of standing or sitting as part of your job or daily life, then find ways to break the monotony every 2 hours. Do this even if it means simply getting up and walking around in your office. It also be as simple as rolling your seat back and bending down to pick up a pen or piece of paper without using a pick up stick or asking for help.

The bottom line is that if you find any exercise pattern that fits into your life style and do it regularly, you will see that daily stress in your life will reduce. The other benefit of daily physical activity is that it can help you increase your daily level of metabolism without making any special effort. On the other hand, if you spend most of your days, sitting in the car, sitting down at work in the office, and sitting down in front of the TV or internet at home, then your daily metabolism will be low and you find yourself gradually gaining more weight.

I am not saying become a weekend warrior and try to build a tree house every weekend. The key emphasis is on simplistic and sustainability. Start with increasing your daily physical activity like mowing your lawn, cleaning your house, washing your car and going for daily walks. Aim for a combined total of about 45 minutes of physical activity most days of the week. Next do not overlook the importance of sleep in helping you lose weight and keep it off.

Assignment

Make increased physical activity part of your daily lifestyle

Write down three more things you could do differently in your daily routine that will help you to become physically more active

Don't be like others who make little effort to sleep better then wonder why they can't lose weight

Sleeping well will help you lose weight and keep it off. As we get older we discover that sleep does not come as readily as in the past. Not sleeping well eventually affects your health. One way most people try to deal with insomnia is to take sleeping pills. However, another option is to increase the amount of physical exercise that you participate in during the day. This is one of the key ways to help you get a good sleep at night. The more active your body is during the day, the more likely you are to relax at night and fall asleep faster.

If you doubt this, watch your children. You will find out they sleep the most, when they have been most busy running around and actively playing all day. They get into bed and fall sound asleep.

With regular exercise you'll notice that your quality of sleep is improved and the transition between the cycles and phases of sleep will become smoother and more regular. By keeping up your physical activity during the day, you may find it easier to deal with the stress and worries of your life.

Research and studies indicate that there is a direct correlation between how much we exercise and how we feel afterwards. You should try and increase your physical activity during the day. The goal here is to give your body enough stimulation during the day so that you aren't full of energy at night.

Your body requires a certain amount of physical activity in order to keep functioning in a healthy manner. It is also important to note that you should not be exercising one or two hours before you go to bed. Make your own individualized time-frame based on your experience.

The ideal exercise time is in the late afternoon or early evening. You want to make sure you expend your physical energy long before it is time for your body to rest and ready itself for sleep.

If you discover that you don't have any time to exercise on a regular basis, you should try to sneak in moments of physical activity into your daily schedule. Whenever possible, you should take the stairs instead of the elevator, and form the habit of walking around whenever it is safe to do so.

Apart from exercise, the other factors that contribute to poor sleep include watching too much TV and using your mobile devices late at night. Don't stay up late to watch your favorite show. You may enjoy your show but you will end up not sleeping well at night. This will not be good for your blood pressure especially if you are over 40 years old. Remember to turn off your computer and your mobile devices like your cell phone and iPad. Your overall goal here is to have a deep and restful sleep of about 6 to 8 hours everyday.

Assignment

Document how many minutes you exercise everyday

Turn off your devices before you go to bed

Make a note of when you get to bed at night and when you wake up

Do you sleep 8 hours every day?

Would like to learn even more ways to make you sleep more?

Improve your emotional well-being

Our emotional well-being is very important for our health because feeling good about ourselves reduces our daily stress level and helps to make our interactions with others more enjoyable. The more stress we have, the more likely it will be that we could suffer from stress overload.

There are factors and activities throughout the day that can affect our emotional well-being. These include time management, money-issues, relationship conflicts, anxiety and anger. The truth is that we all have problems or things we do not do well. Taking part in such activities can lead to emotional tension and stress, unless we learn can manage our emotions well. Our emotions play a big role on how we respond to our daily circumstances. The Compass Method for emotional management encourages us to discover ourselves so that we can manage our emotions in a way that fits our inner self. This is particularly true with different personality types.

According to Linda Malone, people with outgoing personalities like an "I" personality type or sanguine personality, tend to allow stress to accumulate to the point where there response to stress becomes dominated by pleasure-based eating. This is similar to trying to deal with stress by drinking alcohol. It does not work. Pleasure-based eating can lead one to eat too much pleasant tasting food like high-fat content food, and carbohydrate-rich foods like candy and cookies. These two options would lead to high calorie intakes that can lead to weight gain, unless you figure out how to reduce stress, before it triggers excessive eating.

One of the best ways we can protect our emotional well-being and, is to expect the unexpected. Each one of us must find ways to deal with those times when people return kindness with rudeness, fairness with unfairness. Whenever I encounter such situations, I remind myself that how I react is more important than whatever is said by someone else. I begin my "thankful" mantra to help me relax and reduce emotional tension. I purposely become thankful for obvious daily activities like eating, walking, smiling, talking and being able to read small print.

We have to learn how to deal with our social and physical environment. We also have to learn how to interact with others and how we deal with our deepest fears. If we don't get it right, we build up stress that will ultimately affect our sleep, heart and digestive systems. This can lead to sleepless nights and overeating.

We can empower ourselves to deal with such circumstances by reminding yourself that people lash out or say mean things when they feel frustrated, insecure, uncomfortable or unappreciated. This is just an emotional outburst. Do not take such outbursts personal.

Instead treat each outburst or episode as an opportunity to be thankful. Anticipate 5 daily humiliations or toxic emotional outbursts from your interactions with others everyday. One of the ways to empower yourself is to learn your emotional triggers and have strategies to deal with such situations before they arise or as soon as they arise. Self-knowledge, which is one of the seven dimensions of the compass health profile, will definitely enable us to empower ourselves and live more healthy lives. Knowing your DISC personality will help.

While you are in the process of changing these negative patterns that can distort your emotional well-being, create an automatic response that you can use in such situations without having to eat food. My first option in such circumstances is to start an internal dialogue in which I remind myself of the reasons why I am thankful. I then list at least 10 reasons why I am thankful in the present moment. This helps to diffuse emotional tension, reduce stress, and curtail attention seeking bad eating habits. Next make sure you have a strategy for dealing with your daily conflicts.

Assignment

Write down how many emotional outbursts you have encountered today

How did you manage them?

List 10 things you are thankful for today

Don't let your daily conflicts sabotage your stress management strategies

One of the advantages of having an integrated mind set is that it allows you to look at conflicts as an opportunity for change and growth. Conflict resolution is a useful tool for reducing your weight gain because it will help you reduce stress.

Conflicts can teach us a lot about ourselves and how to become more competent and effective in our communications with others. They can also help us avoid relationship minefields because conflicts help each person to recognize behavior patterns that lead to disruptions. Good conflict management can help us eliminate or cut down on stress.

Long standing conflicts indicate a growing need to change and an increasing resistance to doing so.

They expose contradictory social messages and help us to find out when something isn't working and the need for a fresh approach to fix or transcend it. The determining element in reducing stress from daily conflicts, through better management is the mindset of the people involved and their desire to end the conflict.

In a way this is a very sophisticated way of saying that conflicts help us to realize the areas in our lives in which we need to change. To some extent, our conflicts are due to our differing needs, wants, and relationships. The husband might want to spend money and the wife might want to save it. This can lead to misunderstandings and stress build up. The more stress builds up the more you will find yourself taking action that will make you gain weight unless you begin to manage your daily conflicts.

To do this we all need to feel understood and nurtured in our daily encounters with others. The ways we can do this varies broadly because of our different personalities, circumstances, and spiritual outlooks. Recognizing that conflicts are part of every relationship will help us not to take them too personal and use them as opportunities for growth and reduce emotional tension.

How we feel affects how we see ourselves and how we interact with others. If we do not feel good about ourselves, we are less likely to do those things that will make us happy and healthy. For example, being in a bad mood can make us decide to skip the fruits and salads that we know are good for our health. Worse still, you may feel so bad that you end up drinking and smoking. These types of negative behaviors will make it more difficult for you to lose body fat unless we manage our daily conflicts better.

According to a study from the University of Alabama, those who ate in response to an emotional stress- or a daily conflict were 13 times more likely to be overweight or obese. We all know the additional health risks associated with being overweight.

If you are dealing with negative feelings, counter them by finding or saying positive thoughts that will lead to positive feelings and positive action. This will help to resist the urge to drink and splurge on junk food and gain weight. **Next make maintaining balance an important part of your weight loss strategy.**

Assignment

Say 10 positive thoughts everyday

Make maintaining balance an important part of your weight-loss strategy

Balance is an important part of the Compass Method for losing weight and keeping it off. Maintaining the balance that we need to live healthy is not easy for most of us. Although balance is desired, it is hard to achieve. Maintaining daily balance will help you to share your time well between the activities to help you lose weight, your work, and your relationships.

The right balance between your finances, relationships and health will help you to be happy and accomplish your daily goals. When you set your weight loss goals you have to pursue its fulfillment through your desire to succeed and your need for others. After all no man is an island.

We forget that nobody is perfect and fail to maintain the balance between our work and relationships. We sometimes put in 80% of our energy into work, and 20% of our energy into our relationships and we still expect our relationships to be stellar. When our relationships struggle we become frustrated and stressed out.

If we fail to strike the right balance between our work and our relationships then there will be a buildup of stress and illness in our lives. We shall find ourselves quick to anger and less tolerant of others and their mistakes. **We shall find ourselves less able to concentrate and maintain the discipline that will help us to watch what we eat, exercise when we should or let go of daily irritations.**

How much balance do you have in your life? Is your triangle of happiness balanced? To find out how much balance you have in your life spend fifteen minutes of your day, examining how much time you spend on your finances, relationships, and health. How much time do you put into making your weight-loss strategy a priority in your daily life without making other aspects of your life suffer? If you do not strike the right balance and build harmony in your life and environment through your weight-loss strategy, your success will be limited and unsustainable.

This is only the first step in our trying to find balance in our lives. It is an important first step because it allows us to examine our relations, health habits, and finances to determine which aspects require more time and more improvement. Next we focus on ways you can make consistent daily exercise an integral part of your weight-loss strategy.

Assignment

Lower your expectations from others

Forgive and forgive and again

What is your balance time bar chart?

What aspect of your life costs you the most time everyday?

Learn to use consistent daily exercise to help you burn off belly fat

As you get older you begin to notice a tiny but perceptible bulge in your waist line. At first you try to ignore it because you know, you haven't changed your eating habits or daily routine. Yet the bulge continues to grow. Sadly at 40, most people are old enough to notice this type of bulge and increase in waist line. This is usually due to belly fat.

While a few people look at the bulge as a sign good living majority consider it as an embarrassing sign of aging. Knowing why you have the bulge will help you to be more motivated to reduce it. Remember that for men the waist circumference measured above the hip bones while relaxed and exhaling should not be more than 40 inches or

100cm and for women not more than 35 inches or 88cm.The exception is pregnancy for woman.

One of the main reasons why our belly fat increases after 40 is because our muscle mass decreases with age. When this happens our ability to use up energy becomes decreased so that the unused energy becomes converted into visceral fat in our internal organs leading to the belly bulge.

The second reason is that as we get older we have new sources of stress. You now have to worry about your job, your mortgage, your children's education and your in-laws. New sources of stress mean more release of cortisol, the stress hormone. Cortisol leads to the distribution of fat into the abdominal area, making a bad situation worse. Cortisol will also cause the retention of sodium and will lead to increase in water retention and your weight.

Knowing at least these two reasons, you will now look at your belly fat more like a health-marker than as a cosmetic problem and will want to reduce your belly fat fast. Sadly you will discover that the bulge or belly fat is not easy to get rid of. If you have tried to get rid of your own bulge, I am sure you would agree with me.

I will share with you how I lost weight in six weeks, I lost 10 pounds in six weeks by eating plenty of vegetables and fruits while reducing my food portion per meal by about a half and by doing consistent daily exercise. Since I have already discussed the eating part of my plan in the **"adjust your diet" part of this book**, I shall now focus on the exercise part of the plan. I started by walking for at least 45 minutes, at least five times a week. I started by walking 30 minutes a day for the first week, then I increased it to 45 minutes a day. After about 6 weeks, I found it difficult to consistently create the 45 minutes block of time, so

I changed to 3 blocks of 15 minute-time intervals everyday. The advantage of this approach, which is one of the cornerstones of the Compass Method, was that it was gradual and I slowly incorporated it into my lifestyle. It has also helped me to lose fat and become more energetic and active.

To trim your belly fat faster, you need to include exercises that will further strengthen your muscles. This is important because after 40 years of age, muscle strength becomes weaker. If you fail to take action to strengthen your muscles, you will end up with a more protruding belly. You can do this by participating in muscle strengthening activities like playing tennis, walking with extra weights, doing pushups and jump ropes every week. Choose one of these or any other similar one that will work best for your personality, experience and schedule. The key thing is to do whatever you choose regularly and consistently.

I will share with you Ray's method for doing muscle strengthening. Ray is a friend of mine who uses his own unique combination of pushups to tone his muscles. It consists doing at least 50 pushups every day. However, he does it by doing 10 pushups at a time. After each ten, take a 1 to 3 minute break, then continue until you have completed 50 pushups. If you cannot do it all in one session break it up into two or three sessions that you find comfortable. If 50 a day is too high a target for you, start with 20 a day. Do not exceed 50 a day and do you pushups on alternate days, to give your muscles time to recover and grow.

These muscle-strengthening exercises will help you increase your muscle mass as well as increase your total energy expenditure and reduce the amount of excess energy to be converted to visceral or stomach fat. No matter which muscle strengthening exercise you decide to use, take time to warm before you begin to exercise and cool down after exercise. This will help to protect your heart. It is always a good idea to first discuss your exercise plans with your doctor or healthcare professional before you begin. Take time to draw your own weight loss pie chart. It will help you monitor your progress. Next put in place strategies that will help you keep your weight-loss strategy stress-free.

Assignment

Measure your waist circumference

More strategies to keep your weight-loss plan stress-free and able to overcome difficulties

If you want to lose weight in a manner that will last, you have to have strategies that will help make your weight-loss related activities stress-free. If not you will start then stop. Sometimes, I have to chuckle at how we concentrate too much on the total amount of pounds we have to lose, instead of finding simple and easy ways to lose a few pounds per week. In order to lose 23 pounds and keep it off, you have to do it in a way that is fun for you, easy to do and can be made part of your long-term healthy lifestyle.

Once you discover what works for you that you can do consistently, your weight loss will occur naturally. **By following the approaches discussed so far in this book you will discover your own**

individualized plan that is stress-free and easy for you to implement.

First, be realistic do not try to lose 100 pounds in two days or one week. This is very hard to do in an enjoyable and practical manner. Losing weight is not the same as starvation. A more realistic goal might be losing 10 pounds in one month or 6 weeks.

Second, remember the reason why you want to lose weight. Remind yourself of this reason regularly. This has to be the central passion that drives the activities you participate in, everyday to help you lose weight. You already know that you do not want to spend your old age in nursing homes suffering from one chronic illness after another. You want to have fun and age gracefully.

Third, do not worry about results. Concentrate on actually doing or taking the steps you set up in your simple plan for losing weight. If your plan requires walking 45 minutes a day, do it. Do not make excuses. If you are too busy to spare chunks of 45 minutes at a time, then cut it down to 15 minutes at a time.

Fourth, do not think like a child. Do not think that it is either you are getting everything right or everything is wrong. If you plan to walk 45 minutes a day but due to circumstances beyond your control you were able to do only 20 minutes, you have not failed. Do the 20 minutes that day, then do 70 minutes the next day. This still makes a total of 90 minutes in two days. On the third day you can go back to 45 minutes a day. Be flexible.

Fifth, make sure you keep track of your progress. Weigh yourself before you start then weigh yourself after every week. You can use a simple scale to weigh yourself. Measuring your weight regularly is one of the easiest checks on how your individualized health plan is working. It is easier to do than calculating your BMI or measuring your waist circumference. Just climb on a scale and read your weight.

However, If you want something a little more comprehensive, you can calculate your BMI (Body Mass Index), by measuring your height as well. The next step would be to put your height, weight, age and sex, into a BMI calculator and you would find out your BMI. Normal BMI is between 18.5 and 24.9. The advantage of taking measurements is that it gives you an easy way of checking how much progress you have made. When you check that scale and discover that you have actually met your first realistic goal, the smile on your face will encourage you to keep on trying. You will become more energized.

If on the other hand you discover that you have gained back some of the weight you had lost, then do a quick 72 –hour food audit to see the eating patterns that are making you gain weight. Short-term weight gains usually are as a result of increasing calorie intake or eating more food, rather than simply from reducing physical activity.

The last time I discovered I was gaining back some weight through such a review, I discovered that I had a problem with snacks. I eat too much bread at night when I did not feel like sleeping though I needed to be sleeping. This was a bad idea and I only find out early because I had formed the habit of weighing myself every week. I was able to catch my weight gain and go back to my own individualized plan for weight loss. I replaced the late night snacks with small portions of nuts and banana.

A lapse is not a relapse. A mistake is not a failure. If you find yourself not sticking to your fruits and vegetables, think about trying out new fruits that you have not tried in the past. Talk to your support group, and share your ideas on eating time and food variety. Try again if you do not succeed the first time. If you are living by yourself and are longer in touch with your family or old friends, create a new support group or join one online. Become more active in your community. Volunteer in the church or other societies that you belong to.

Finally, do not forget to talk to your doctor or health care provider about your medications. Make sure you are not taking any medications that may make you gain weight. This is particularly important if through a chart of your weekly weight measurement you discover you have either been gaining weight or not losing as much as you expected.

Losing weight and maintaining your weight within the normal range for your age and height is certainly one of the ways to protect your health and prevent yourself from potentially deadly health complications like heart attacks. Next join a group or share your concerns with one. You don't have to go it alone.

Assignment

Weigh yourself every week

Find out or calculate your BMI

Take advantage of a group to make your weight-loss strategy easier

Do not try to do everything by yourself. Join a group or form one. This is because no man is an island. It does not have to be a formal group. It could easily be a group made up of family members or friends. Believe me, it is a lot of fun when the whole family is involved in healthy eating and healthy living activities like running and sports events or meets.

Making everybody in your family a part of your healthy living plan is a great idea. If you tell your children that you are no longer going to drink soda with your meals, they will remind you if you forget and try to do it. They will keep you accountable.

Another benefit, you get out of this, is that you start getting into the act of eating healthy. It will be easier to buy milk with reduced fat and get the whole family to eat small carrots and pomegranates.

The next people you need to get into your group will be those in your office whom you share a lunch break with. This way when you think of going for soda, candies and cookies, you will have someone reminding you that you have decided to eat fruits and vegetables during your lunch break. A salad is also a good way to go.

Depending on your budget and personality, you may want to try more formal groups than the ones I have mentioned above. These may be online or offline groups. Whatever group you decide to join, make sure you join a group that suits your personality, your budget and your time.

One major advantage of joining a physical group or becoming part of an online community of people trying to lose weight, is that other people can support you. This can be done by helping you to become more accountable to yourself and others. This can be through reminding you to do your exercise, weigh yourself or even discussing challenges and solutions with a mentor or other group members. Next have a financial plan that will help you carry out your weight loss strategy.

Assignment

Join either a physical group or sign up online to a weight loss membership site or forum

Find out about local running events or sports tournaments in your city and participate in those that interest you

Have a financial plan that will help you to reduce your weight and protect your health

If you do not have a financial plan that will help you to protect your health, you will end up with financial stress that will make it impossible for you to lose weight and keep it off. We have to remember that we need money to buy healthy food, to participate in sports activities, go to the laboratory for tests or doctor's visits, and go to the movies.

Not having finances to pay your rent or your mortgage could quickly build up your stress level. You have to remember that no matter the source of stress, whether it is physical, physiological or psychological, chronic stress will eventually lead to damage to your heart, vessels and other organs.

Poor coping mechanisms for coping with stress eventually lead to overeating and weight gain.

This is one of the reasons why it is important that when you are examining your ambition and self-knowledge profile, you should be try as much as possible to estimate how much you earn and how you will spend it. Remember that if you are retired, there is a fixed income, you get every month. Plan your budget accordingly and be selective on how you spend your money.

The state of your finances or unstable financial situation could significantly affect your ability to implement your individualized compass health plan. If you do not have enough money to buy fruits, vegetables, and nuts, you will end up buying mostly cheap calorie-dense processed foods.

One way to make your money go further would be to get all the preventive cares your insurance covers. Ask questions so that you will remain fully informed. Secondly set up a good financial plan. At least having a financial plan will help you to reduce the stress that comes from not knowing what to do. This in turn will help to reduce the level of stress hormones in your body. The less stress hormones you have, the less belly fat you will have. The less fat you accumulate in your internal organs, the more you protect your health. Next we shall look at some of the recurrent challenges and their potential solutions, as you continue on your weight-loss journey.

Assignment

Have a third pathway independent financial plan

Find out from your insurance all the free routine services that they cover for you

Shop at your local farmer's market regularly

Challenges and solutions

In the face of cravings for more food between meals, snack with nuts. Eat almonds which can make you feel full quickly. This is a common challenge when you first begin trying to adjust your meal to lose weight.

When you do not feel like going outside to exercise, do it inside. Try to be consistent with a little daily exercise, even if you cannot do as much exercise as you would like to. **The Compass Method for sustainable weight loss is based on your ability to form sustainable new healthy habits. It is better to keep on moving at a slow pace, than to stop or give up.**

If after the initial quick weight loss, the remaining pounds begin to prove more difficult, continue to make adjustments. Repeat your food audit, to find out if you have not unwittingly started eating more. Make sure you do not have any underlying medical condition that could be making you gain weight or that your weight gain is not the side effect of one of your medications.

The other reason why people gain weight after an initial loss of weight is that they cut down on physical activity. **Make sure you have not become too busy to protect your health**. If you have stopped using your treadmill, it is not too late, begin again. If doing it by yourself is too boring, partner up. Join a group or join an online membership site for weight loss. This will help you become more accountable.

Change takes time, be patient. Communicate better. Write down goals that are specific, measurable, attainable, and time dependent. Even if you do not accomplish them at your first attempt, try again.

Reduce stress by talking strategically with others. Take a deep breath, sleep well and begin everyday with discipline and renewed determination despite challenges and doubts. Remember that the journey of a thousand miles begins with the first step, but ends with the last step on the thousandth mile. In order to lose weight and keep it off, you have to be able to begin and preserve to the end. **Don't be afraid to ask questions, share concerns, problems and successes. Growth is a process.**

Daily action tips

UNDERSTAND YOURSELF BETTER

KNOW YOUR PASSION

LEARN YOUR DISC PERSONALITY

DO A 72-HOUR FOOD AUDIT

CUT DOWN YOUR SERVING PORTIONS

EAT FOOD RICH IN FRUITS AND WHOLE GRAINS

MODIFY YOUR TYPICAL CULTURAL FOOD

DRINK TWO GLASSES OF WATER BEFORE EVERY MEAL

PLAN FOR YOUR SNACKS

CUTDOWN ON SODA AND BEER

READ YOUR NUTRITION FACTS

REDUCE SODIUM INTAKE

REDUCE SUGAR INTAKE

FOCUS ON EATING AND EAT SLOWLY

MANAGE YOUR CONVERSATIONS: YOU DON'T HAVE TO HAVE THE LAST WORD

EXERCISE EVERYDAY:

WALK 4 MILES EVERY DAY

SLEEP WELL

TURN OFF YOUR DEVICES

IMPROVE YOUR EMOTIONAL WELL-BEING

IGNORE EMOTIONAL OUTBURSTS

LOWER YOUR EXPECTATIONS FROM OTHERS

FORGIVE AND FORGIVE AGAIN

FIND AND SAY 10 THANKFUL AND POSITIVE THOUGHTS EVERYDAY

MEASURE YOUR WAIST CIRCUMFERENCE

FIND OUT OR CALCULATE YOUR BMI

A LAPSE IS A NOT A RELAPSE

WEIGH YOURSELF EVERY WEEK

HAVE A THIRD-PATHWAY INDEPENDENT FINANCIAL PLAN

BECOME PART OF A GROUP OR A TEAM

Appendix

BMI=Body mass index. It is a way of assessing your weight and its associated health risks.

DEVELOP YOUR OWN INDIVIDUALIZED BLUE PRINT FOR LOSING WEIGHT AND KEEPING IT OFF

If you have any questions contact me through www.compasswellnessinstitute.com

What will you do if your diet adjustment strategy fails or you cannot sustain your daily exercise regimen?

Do not give up. Reduce it to what you can do. If you cannot walk 4 miles a day, start with 1 mile a day. Build up slowly.

If you cannot cut down your food portion by half, cut it down by a quarter or by a third.

Add fruits and nuts slowly while you reduce your sodium and sugar intake.

Remember that sustainable change is a slow process. Do not give up on yourself. Don't forget to always consult your doctor and keep your appointments.

Notes

American Heart Association

American Journal of Clinical Nutrition

Anshel, M. H. (2010). The disconnected values (intervention) model for promoting healthy habits in religious institutions. *Journal of Religion and Health, 49*(1), 32-49. doi: http://dx.doi.org/10.1007/s10943-008-9230-x

Bermudez, O. I., Gao, X. (2011, January). Greater consumption of sweetened beverages and added sugars is associated with obesity among US young adults. *Annals of Nutrition & Metabolism,* 57(3-4) 211-8

Boyle, M.A. & Long, S. (2010) Personal

Nutrition. Belmont, CA. Wadsworth
Cengage learning

CDC(2015)Division of nutrition, physical
activity and obesity: Adult obesity facts.
Retrieved from
http://www.cdc.gov/obesity/data/adult.ht
ml

Cleland, V.J., Schmidt , M.D., Dwyer, T., &
Venn, A.J. (2008,May).Television viewing
and abdominal obesity in young adults:
is the association mediated by food and
beverage consumption during viewing
time or reduced leisure-time physical
activity? *The American Journal of
Clinical Nutrition, 87*(5).

Daniels, K., & Archibald, P. (2011). The

levitical cycle of health: The church as a public health social work conduit for health promotion. *Social Work and Christianity, 38*(1), 88-100.

Feist, J., & Feist, G. J. (2009). Theories of Personality (7th ed.). New York: McGraw-Hill.

Melone, L.(2014). Healthy living: 10 ways your personality affects your weight. *Huff Post* online publication.

Nutrition Research

Reuters Health (2013).Despite obesity rise, US calories intake trending downwards. Retrieved from http://www.reuters.com/article/2013/03/06/us-despite-obesity-rise-idUSBRE92518620130306

Samaranayake, N. R., Ong, K. L., Raymond,

Y.H. L.,& Chueng, B. M.Y., (2012,May).
Management of obesity in the national
health and nutrition examination survey
(NHANES), 2007–2008. *Annals of
Epidemiology, 22(5),349-353*.

Resources

Here are additional resources that will help you live a healthy, happy and successful life.

www.compasswellnessinstitute.com

www.compasshealthtransformer.com/members

www.dcompassmarketing.com

www.amenfathermbaka.com

http://www.amazon.com/Dr.-Chio-Ugochukwu/e/B00JNFLPQQ

Other books by Dr. Chio Ugochukwu that will help you improve your health, reduce stress and transform your life include;

The Compass Health Transformer: Your 72 Hour Blue Print For Healthy Living

21 Ways To Transform Your Health Without Medications

"…21 simple proven ways to reduce stress and improve your health and wellbeing without relying on medications. These are easy and effective ways you can use to turn your daily challenges into transformative opportunities for healthy living and daily happiness. You can start right away without spending a fortune!.."

Get your own copy of 21 Ways To Transform Your Health Without Medications

The Compass Health Transformer Quit Smoking

Overcoming Daily Stress: 21 Quick And Easy Ways To Stay Stress-Free In Your Daily Life

"…Are you tired of being stressed out everyday? Are you tired of feeling exhausted and overwhelmed in your daily activities? Are you fed up with communication issues in your relationship? Here are 21 quick and easy ways you can use to overcome daily stress and turn your daily challenges into opportunities for transformative abundant living. This book will help you gain a better understanding of your potential communication issues, daily 'stress points' and the steps you can take to overcome them…".

Get your own copy of Overcoming Daily Stress

The Secret To Daily happiness

"..Have you ever wondered why daily happiness has continued to elude you? Do you want to make sustainable daily happiness part of your life? By reading this book. you can find answers to these questions and many more on how to overcome the many obstacles and challenges that daily try to take away your inner peace and contentment…"

Get your own copy of The Secret To Happiness

15 Simple Ways to lower your blood pressure naturally after 40 without complicated diets

"……Don't spend your most productive years dealing with high blood pressure, medications and side effects. Stop worrying about whether you forgot to take your first medication or the second one. Take these simple steps to lower your blood pressure naturally and minimize your need for multiple medications. Did you know that high blood pressure can cause heart attack, stroke, kidney failure, blindness and memory problems? Don't wait to find out! Take Action! ,,,,,"

Click Here for Your own copy of 15 Simple Ways To Reduce Blood Pressure....

Prating To Win: How To Get More Victories And Riches In Your Daily Life Through Spiritual Principles

"..You too can achieve your goals and dreams, through praying to win. You can do this by immersing yourself in the word of God and transforming the moments that make up your daily life through persistent adoration……. Above all, thank God everyday, never give up and persistently continue praying to win..."

Get your own copy of Praying To Win

Managing Time For Success

Too Young To Die

"A book about coping with grief and finding your way in life…"

To order new or additional copies, please visit:

http://www.amazon.com/Dr.-Chio-Ugochukwu/e/B00JNFLPQQ

Call: 661 992 6436

You can also get EBOOKS from

www.compasswellnessinstitute.com/Ebooks

About the Author

Dr. Chio Ugochukwu has always been interested in helping people improve their health, reduce stress, transform their lives, and become the best versions of themselves. He created the Transformational Abundant Living System (TALS) and developed the Compass Method to help individuals stay healthy and become more. He founded the Compass Research Institute to help individuals and organizations, maximize their strengths and overcome their weaknesses to get the best performance out of themselves, and become more empowered in their search for better health, more success and greater happiness despite their busy schedules, daily activities and duties.

He was inspired to create the TALS and the Compass Method, through the challenges he has encountered in his journey of life, his practice of medicine and his fascination with how the mind, the spirit and human experience influence the fulfillment of life. TALS is available at www.compasswellnessinstitute.com.

As an author and researcher, he has published many books, with peer-reviewed publications on quality of life and numerous articles on transformational living. He is the medical director of Dala Compass Foundation and a consultant with the Compass Research Institute. As a life-long learner, He is focused on sharing with individuals and organizations, customized methods and strategic pathways for improving health and getting the best performance for themselves and their organizations.

www.ingramcontent.com/pod-product-compliance
Lightning Source LLC
Chambersburg PA
CBHW060109300526
45791CB00018B/593